✓ **W9-DAL-863**

Live Better colour therapy

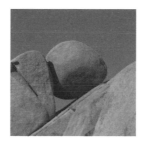

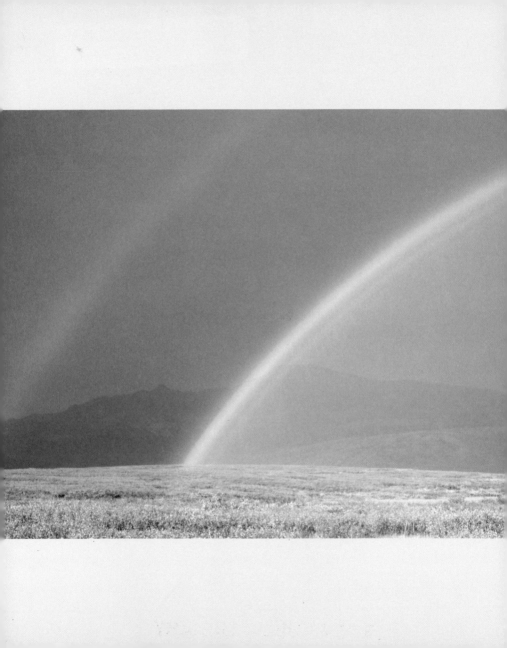

Live Better colour therapy

therapies and techniques for well-being

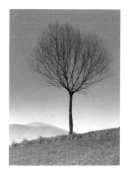

Pauline Wills

DUNCAN BAIRD PUBLISHERS

LONDON

Live Better: colour therapy
Pauline Wills

First published in the United Kingdom and
Ireland in 2006 by
Duncan Baird Publishers Ltd
Sixth Floor
Castle House
75–76 Wells Street
London W1T 3QH

Conceived, created and designed by Duncan
Baird Publishers

Managing Editor: Grace Cheetham
Editor: James Hodgson
Managing Designer: Manisha Patel
Designer: Sailesh Patel
Picture Researcher: Julia Ruxton

British Library Cataloguing-in-Publication Data:
A CIP record for this book is available from the
British Library

ISBN-10: 1-84483-239-2
ISBN-13: 9-781844-832392

10 9 8 7 6 5 4 3 2 1

Typeset in Filosofia and Son Kern
Colour reproduction by Scanhouse, Malaysia
Printed by Imago Singapore

Publisher's note

Before following any advice or practice
suggested in this book, it is recommended
that you consult your doctor as to its
suitability, especially if you suffer from
any health problems or special conditions.
The publishers and author cannot accept
any responsibility for injuries or damage
incurred as a result of using any of the
techniques described or mentioned herein.

contents

INTRODUCTION

Wherever we are, whatever we're doing, colour is with us every second of our lives. Even when we sleep, colour appears in our dreams. But what few of us realize is that throughout our lives our own personal electromagnetic field, the aura (see page 24), cloaks each of us with a vibrant array of ever-changing colours determined by our thoughts, emotions and physical condition.

We may, therefore, call ourselves beings of light, surrounded and interpenetrated as we are by the colours that constitute light. Each colour has its own spectrum of hues and tints and its own vibrational frequencies, which can be measured scientifically. Colour therapy involves identifying and administering the specific colour combinations we need to maintain physical, mental and emotional equilibrium. In this way we can stay healthy and help ourselves to find and deal with the cause of any problems we might be experiencing.

Colour's ability to affect our body, mind and spirit, gives it the power to calm, excite, inspire, balance, bring about a state of harmony and to heal. It even possesses a language of its own. How many times have you heard or used expressions such as "green with envy", "red with anger", "feeling blue", "white as a sheet" or "looking off colour"? To a colour therapist, being "off colour" means either that certain colours are missing from our aura or that colours are appearing in the wrong place.

This book will give you some insight into the wonderful world of colour. It will introduce you to the history of colour therapy and how it has been used in various cultures; it will explain the attributes of the individual colours that make up the aura's ever-changing cloak, and it will show the various ways in which you can harness the healing energies of these colours to address disorders and imbalances.

As you practise the exercises and visualizations contained within this book, you will find yourself gradually becoming aware of, and sensitive to, colour's vibrational energies, enabling you to realize the colour you need at any given time to help you to develop and maintain a sense of calm, joy and well-being.

what is colour?

For centuries, no one knew why the rainbow arched across the sky after a storm or why its colours always appeared in the same order. It was long believed that the colours were produced by differing mixtures of light and darkness. However, in 1666 the English scientist Sir Isaac Newton discovered that the colours of the spectrum were, in fact, all contained in white light. In a darkened room, he passed a ray of light through a prism. He found that the prism refracted the light and, because each colour has a different angle of refraction, a rainbow of colours emerged from the opposite side of the prism. The appearance of a rainbow is the result of raindrops acting like a prism, refracting the sunlight. The larger the rain-drops, the purer and brighter the refracted colours.

Each colour of the spectrum vibrates at its own frequency and has its own wavelength. Albert Einstein proved that the spectral colours are composed of small packets of energy, which he called photons. The longer the wavelength the more spaced out the pho-tons. The colours blue, indigo and violet have short wavelengths and compacted photons, and so contain the most energy. The colours at the other end of the spectrum have longer wavelengths and less energy.

In this chapter, we will look in more detail at colour energy, which lies at the heart of colour therapy.

THE IMPORTANCE OF COLOUR

The vibrational energies of colour contained in sunlight are essential for our health – indeed, no life form could survive without the light and warmth of the sun. In the summer, when we tend to spend more time outdoors, most of us feel happier and healthier.

One condition resulting from light deprivation is Seasonal Affective Disorder (SAD). This begins in autumn, when days become shorter and our exposure to sunlight is diminished, and disappears in spring as the days lengthen again. The symptoms of SAD are lethargy, depression and a craving for carbohydrates.

Sunlight also helps to build strong, healthy bones. When we spend time outdoors, we absorb through our eyes the middle waveband of ultraviolet light, which enables the body to produce vitamin D, essential for the metabolization of calcium. Researchers have shown that ultraviolet light cannot pass through glass, so wearing spectacles, sunglasses (particularly of the "wraparound" variety) or contact lenses inhibits its absorption.

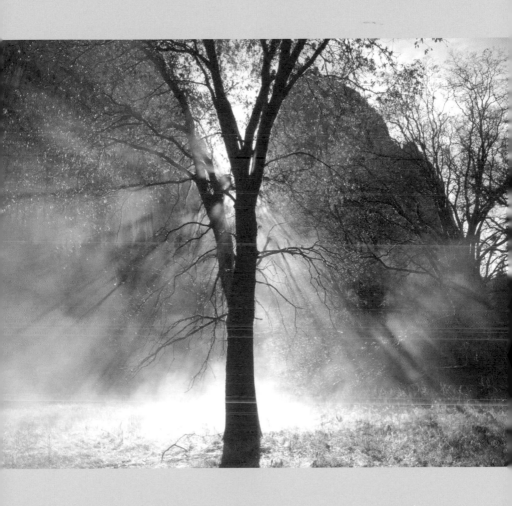

THE HISTORY OF COLOUR THERAPY

In his books on the lost city of Atlantis, Frank Alper attributes to the Atlanteans the earliest use of colour therapy. He describes circular temples containing heal- ing rooms. Roofs of interlocking crystals refracted the sunlight, filling the rooms with the spectral colours. These chambers were used not only for treating ail- ments, but for aiding childbirth and helping the dying to make the transition from earthly to spiritual life.

Archaeologists have discovered that the Egyptians, too, had healing rooms built into their temples – rooms constructed so that when sunlight entered them its rays were separated into the colours of the spectrum. Patients were "colour diagnosed", then treated in the room that radiated the prescribed colour.

In ancient India, medical treatment included the use of minerals and gemstones, which were believed to be a concentration of the seven cosmic rays – each stone relating to a certain ray (for example, onyx to ultraviolet, cat's eye to infrared). Healers viewed the gems through a prism to ascertain their true cosmic colour, which was not always the same as their manifested colour.

Among the ancient Greeks, treatment by sunlight (heliotherapy) was a common practice, the city of Heliopolis being famous for its healing temples. The physician Hippocrates explained the basic mechanism of illness in terms of four humours or bodily fluids, each of which was designated by a different colour. These were red blood, connected to the heart; yellow bile, associated with the spleen; black bile, arising in the brain; and white phlegm, deriving from the liver. Good health required these four humours to be kept in equilibrium – imbalances were remedied by administering the colour of the deficient humour in the form of food, flowers, plasters, ointments and minerals.

During the early Christian era, medical practices involving colour were deemed to be pagan, and many of the ancient writings on holistic medicine have been lost. Colour therapy was revived in the eleventh century CE by an outstanding Persian physician named Avicenna. His most famous book, *The Canon*, sets out his theories on

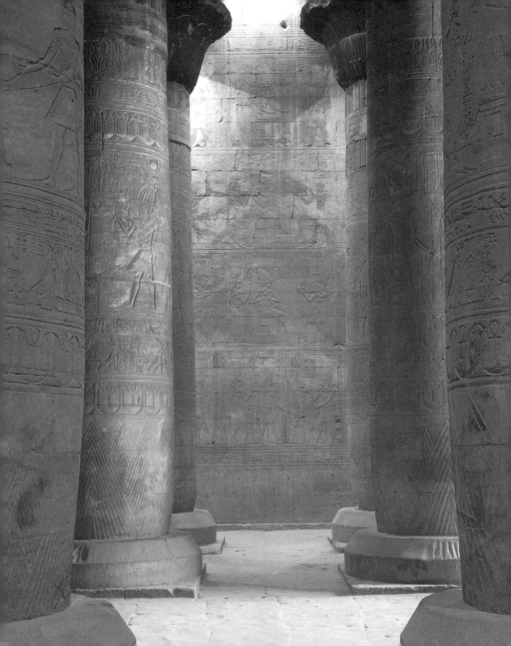

the therapeutic use of colour – including the adverse effects that colour can produce. For example, he noted that red increased blood pressure and blue lowered it, while yellow seemed to reduce inflammation and pain.

In Renaissance Europe, another notable physician, named Paracelsus, medicated with colour, which he administered in the form of light, herbs and minerals.

In the nineteenth century there were great advances in the understanding of anatomy, surgery and medication. This emphasis on the physical marginalized the spiritual, emotional and psychological aspects of healing, and the concept of treating the whole person was lost. With this loss the use of colour therapy declined.

However, heliotherapy was rediscovered in the mid-nineteenth century. The Danish physician Niels Ryberg Finsen was the first to use artificial light to treat skin tuberculosis. In Switzerland, Augustus Rollier used heliotherapy on a larger scale both to prevent and to treat tuberculosis.

Practitioners of heliotherapy now began to turn their attention to the colours that make up sunlight. Pioneers included the American physicians Seth Pancoast and Edwin Babbit. Pancoast worked mainly with red and blue, believing that the red ray accelerated the nervous system and the blue ray relaxed it. Babbit's work involved the red, yellow and blue primaries. He encouraged his patients to drink colour-solarized water, and also invented a cabinet, which he called the "Thermolume", to administer coloured sunlight.

In the early twentieth century, the philosopher, mystic and teacher Rudolf Steiner considered colour from a metaphysical point of view. He believed that colour was a living entity, each hue bearing a spiritual significance. He argued that illness was caused by the separation of earthly consciousness from higher perception, and that we could heal this rift through art.

Max Lüscher, a professor of psychology from Basle University, contended that by measuring a person's preference for certain colours it was possible to diagnose and treat both physical and psychological conditions. Lüscher's colour theories were supported by a Russian scientist S.V. Krakov, who later proved that red stimulates the sympathetic nervous system, which accelerates autonomic (involuntary) body functions, such as breathing and heartbeat, while blue stimulates the parasympathetic system, which slows them down.

Two further twentieth-century colour therapy innovators were Dinshah P. Ghadiali and Harry Riley Spitler. Ghadiali, well versed in electricity, mathematics and physics, argued that sound, light, colour and heat were all the same energy, only differentiated from each other by their vibrational frequency. He formulated a scientific approach for the application of colour to the human body, inventing two machines designed to apply, through slides, the 12 colours with which he worked. Spitler, a medical doctor and optometrist, was responsible for a system of colour treatment which he called "Syntonics". He demonstrated that light entering the eyes plays an important role in the functioning of both the endocrine and autonomic nervous systems.

The colour therapy of today benefits from the influence of these enquiring minds and continues to develop, as we shall see in this book.

COLOUR AND LIGHT IN
CONVENTIONAL MEDICINE

Although commonly seen as the tools of complementary therapy, colour and light are also used in modern allopathic medicine. For example, skin problems such as acne and psoriasis can be treated with ultraviolet light. In surgery, the argon laser, which produces the green wavelength, is used to stem bleeding tissues; the carbon dioxide laser, which produces an infrared beam, is used to make incisions. In ophthalmology, lasers are used to treat detached retinas and proliferative retinopathy.

Soft laser light, pioneered by Professor Endre Mester, alleviates burn pain, accelerates the healing of wounds and reduces scar tissue. Hungarian scientists have developed polarized light treatment to heal leg ulcers and bedsores, and to deal with varicose veins.

Two forms of treatment being carried out in Russia by Professor Kira Samoilova are Ultraviolet Irradiated Blood Retransfusions (UVIBR) and Intravenous Visible Light Irradiation of Blood (ILIB). These techniques were built upon research initially carried out by Emmitt Knott and Virgil Hancock. Dr Knott invented an instrument called the Haemo-Irradiation Machine, which irradiated with ultraviolet light a small sample of a patient's blood – blood which was then reinfused into the patient. The published findings of Knott and Hancock included accounts of the successful treatment, by this method, of viral infections, peritonitis and advanced toxaemia – treatment that worked where conventional drug therapy had failed. The treatment was used in Germany, the United States and the Soviet Union until the mid-1950s. It was then abandoned until the mid-1970s when it was reintroduced into medicine in the Soviet Union.

Another important treatment, pioneered in the United States in 1970 by Thomas Dougherty, is called Photodynamic Therapy (PDT). This technique uses red light, in conjunction with a light-sensitive compound, to eliminate malignant tumours. Doctors have also used PDT to treat skin cancer and to reduce scarring at the site from which a malignant tumour has been removed.

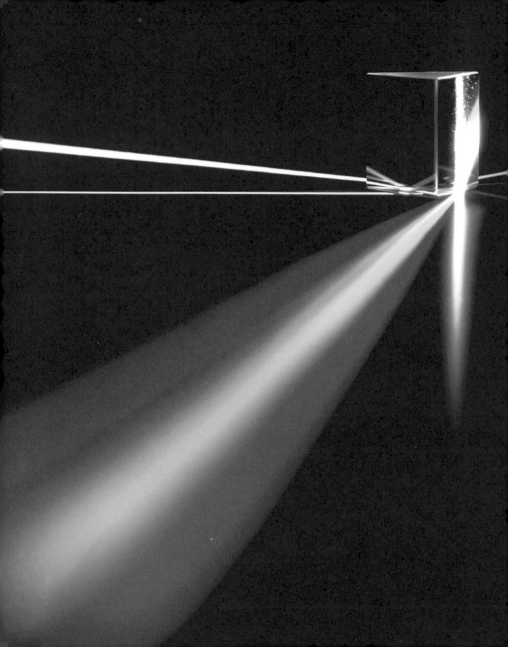

HOW WE SEE COLOUR

Light is colour and colour is light. There are no actual colours in the world around us – only the waves, of varying lengths, which constitute light. These waves are absorbed and reflected by everything that light hits. The reflected waves enter our eyes, activating the rod and cone cells situated at the back of the eye, on the retina. These then transmit the light-triggered signals, via the optic nerve, to the visual centre at the back of the brain. It is only when this has occurred that we "see" colour.

When light enters our eyes, it facilitates the healthy functioning of the body by having a direct influence on the hypothalamus. The hypothalamus serves as our biological clock, controlling the nervous system and stimulating our hormonal system through the light information it sends to the pineal gland.

To experience the colours present in light, you need a prism. If you place the prism on the bridge of your nose and look through it at the objects around you, you will see around each one the colours of the spectrum.

THE ELECTROMAGNETIC SPECTRUM

The diagram of the electromagnetic spectrum, opposite, shows the electromagnetic energy emanating from the sun, from the longest waves (radio waves) to the shortest (cosmic rays). Wavelengths are measured in nanometres (one nanometre is equivalent to one billionth of a metre). Much of the electromagnetic spectrum is invisible to the human eye, but that doesn't mean that these unseeable rays have no effect on us. For example, X-ray machines are an indispensable diagnostic tool in conventional medicine, and ultraviolet light provides us with vitamin D (see page 10). However, the effects can also be harmful: over-exposure to ultraviolet rays causes sunburn and can lead to skin cancer.

In the centre of the electromagnetic spectrum, with wavelengths ranging from around 400 to around 700 nanometres, lie the waves of light that are visible to us and that provide us with colour. Like all the other rays, they are a form of radiation and can therefore affect us in subtle ways, as we shall see.

SHORT WAVES

Cosmic rays

Gamma rays

X-rays

Ultraviolet rays

VISIBLE LIGHT

Infrared rays

Radio waves

LONG WAVES

THE HUMAN AURA

All living things are surrounded by their own electro-magnetic field, known as an aura. In humans, the aura is egg-shaped — wider around the head and narrower around the feet. It comprises six layers or sheaths which penetrate each other and our body. Each layer vibrates at a different frequency, which determines the interplay of colours within it. The colours in the layers relating to the physical body are dense and vibrant whereas the colours in the sheaths representing a person's spiritual aspects are more ethereal. The colours and the vibrational frequency of each of the aural layers change with our thoughts and feelings. These changes ultimately affect our physical well-being either positively or negatively.

The aura is a living part of the self and it constantly expands and contracts. How far it expands depends upon our spiritual growth. Man-made fibres appear to interfere with these expansions and contractions: for this reason it is best to choose only natural fibres if you are using materials as colour filters.

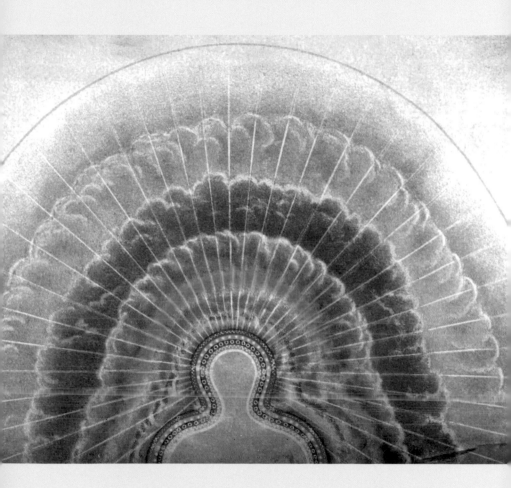

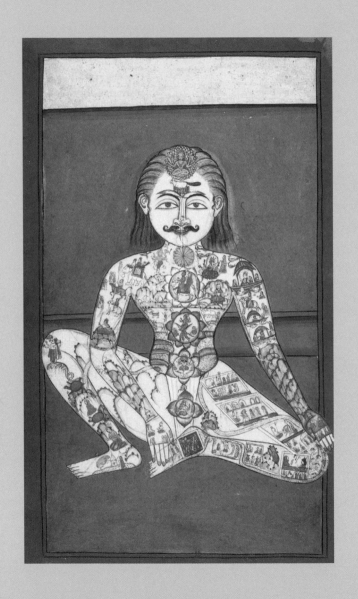

THE MAJOR CHAKRAS

Chakras (from the Sanskrit for "wheel") are focal points where the energies contained within the aura are received by the physical body and distributed within it. Traditional Hindu belief holds that there are seven major chakras (see pages 28–29), located in a line running up the centre of the body from the base of the spine to the crown. Another important chakra is the Alta Major Chakra (see page 29). Each of these eight chakras is connected to one of our endocrine glands, which secrete hormones directly into the bloodstream (opinions vary as to which gland is linked with which chakra).

The chakras work in harmony with each other, and each of the seven traditional chakras radiates to the frequency of one of the spectral colours. If any one of the chakras malfunctions, the whole system becomes imbalanced, which blocks energy flow through our body and jeopardizes our well-being. As well as disciplines such as yoga and meditation, the application of appropriate colour can help to rebalance our chakra system.

Below is a summary of the properties of each of the major chakras, including the Alta Major Chakra:

Base Chakra Situated at the base of the spine, the Base Chakra radiates the colour red. It relates to the earth element and the sense of smell. It influences our blood, spine, legs, bones and nervous system, as well as the vagina (in women), and is linked with the testes (in men).

Sacral Chakra Lying just below the navel, the Sacral Chakra radiates orange. It is connected to the water element and the sense of taste. It influences the female reproductive organs, mammary glands, kidneys and skin, and its associated endocrine glands are the adrenals.

Solar Plexus Chakra Found just above the navel, this chakra radiates yellow. It is associated with fire and the sense of sight. It influences skin and digestion and is linked to the endocrine system via the islets of langerhans.

Heart Chakra Slightly to the right of the physical heart, the Heart Chakra is related to the colour green and to the air element and the sense of touch. It influences the heart and lungs, as well as the immune and circulatory systems, and it is associated with the thymus gland.

Throat Chakra This chakra is situated in the region of the throat, between the collarbones. It radiates the colour blue and is connected to the element ether and the sense of hearing. Physically, it affects our throat, neck, ears and shoulders. The Throat Chakra's associated endocrine gland is the thyroid.

Brow Chakra Found on the forehead, midway between the eyebrows, the Brow Chakra radiates indigo. It relates to the brain, eyes, ears and nose, and the nervous system. Its associated endocrine gland is the pituitary.

Crown Chakra Located just above the head and radiating the colour violet, the Crown Chakra governs the brain and the nervous system. It is connected to the endocrine system through the pineal gland.

Alta Major Chakra This important chakra is sometimes known as "the mouth of God" because it is here that life force is channelled into the physical body. It is located in the medulla oblongata, at the base of the brain, and continues into the spinal cord. The Alta Major Chakra radiates white and is connected with the carotid glands in the neck.

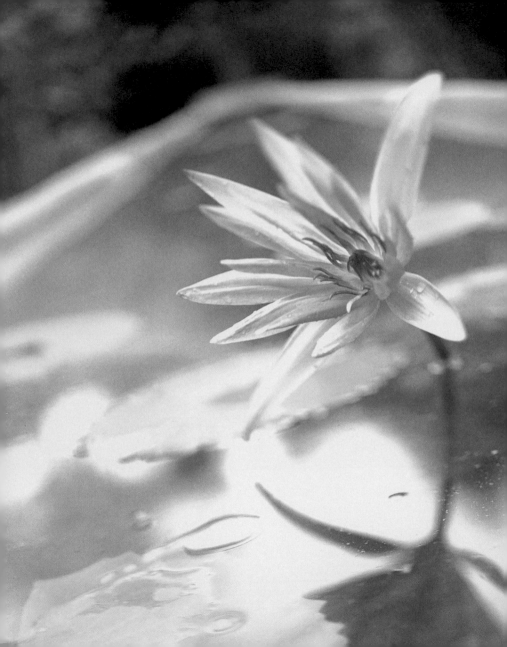

To keep the body in good health is a duty, for otherwise
we shall not be able to trim the lamp of wisdom,
and keep our mind strong and clear.
Water surrounds the lotus flower,
but does not wet its petals.

THE BUDDHA

(563–483 BC)

THE HEALING POWER OF COLOUR

Colour is a living energy which affects us profoundly on all levels of our being. How many times have you walked through a wood carpeted with bluebells or over a vivid green lawn and felt your spirits being lifted? No one has been able to provide a cast-iron scientific explanation of why diferent colours affect our emotions in different ways. One theory is that the way in which light, having entered the eye, interacts with the hypothalamus, and the endocrine secretions that it triggers (see page 21), are influenced by the particular colours that we see.

The aura surrounds and penetrates us with the vibrational frequencies of colour (see page 24). These are constantly changing. When we are unwell it is because parts of the aura either are vibrating at the wrong colour frequency or are devoid of colour. The problem starts in the aura and, if not rectified at this level, it will eventually manifest as a physical disease. The physical body can therefore be seen as a mirror that reflects our emotional, mental and spiritual states.

Using colour frequencies to bring us back into a state of well-being is a very powerful tool, because we are working with our basic nature as beings of light. Colour healing requires the administration of the correct colour frequencies, using either light or pigment. Of these two, light has the more profound effect upon cellular structure and, for this reason, is used therapeutically by qualified colour practitioners. However, because of light's powerful effect upon us through its ability to alter our biochemical structure, and because some colours can have contra-indications, it is not advisable to attempt this method on yourself.

Colour is used to treat physical disease by promoting a state of balance in the sufferer. It is also used to help individuals find and then deal with the cause of the underlying imbalance. This process, together with counselling, is a vital part of any therapy, for if the source of the imbalance is not addressed its physical symptoms will recur. When the cause has been acknowledged, it is then up to the individual to decide whether he or she is willing to take the necessary steps to deal with it.

ADDITIVE AND SUBTRACTIVE COLOUR

Newton demonstrated that when all the colours of the spectrum are combined they produce white light. Later research showed that adding together just the three spectral primaries – red, green and blue – will produce white light and, with various permutations, all possible spectral colours. When rays of colour are combined in this way they form what are known as additive colours.

However, when dyes or paints are mixed, or when transparent coloured filters are superimposed on each other, the colours obtained are the result of the subtraction of certain colours from the light passing through the combined pigments. Whereas a mixture of the three additive primaries produces white light, the three subtractive primaries – cyan, yellow and magenta – combine to produce an approximation of black.

Some colour therapists use subtractive colours to produce the "wheel" of 12 colours with which they treat their patients. However, the choice and number of colours varies from one practitioner to another.

ADDITIVE COLOUR

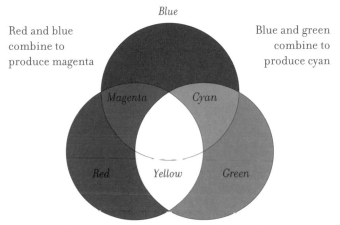

Blue

Red and blue
combine to
produce magenta

Blue and green
combine to
produce cyan

Magenta   Cyan

Red   Yellow   Green

Green and red combine to produce yellow

SUBTRACTIVE COLOUR

In the notes to this diagram, we focus on cyan and its two secondary colours. The same principles apply to magenta and yellow.

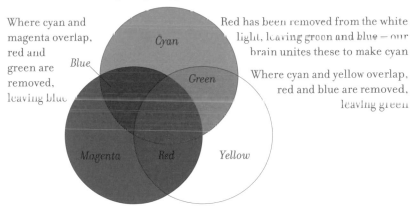

Where cyan and
magenta overlap,
red and
green are
removed,
leaving blue

Cyan

Blue

Green

Magenta   Red   Yellow

Red has been removed from the white
light, leaving green and blue – our
brain unites these to make cyan

Where cyan and yellow overlap,
red and blue are removed,
leaving green

Where all three circles overlap, red, green
and blue are removed, obliterating all light

MAKING A 12-COLOUR WHEEL

When the three subtractive primaries, yellow, magenta and cyan, are mixed together in pairs they produce the subtractive secondary colours, red, blue and green. A primary colour can then be mixed with each of its flanking secondaries to produce a 12-colour wheel.

The drawback with such a wheel is that it doesn't contain indigo or gold, two colours that I consider to be very important in therapy. The 12-colour wheel that I use (see opposite) is based on red, blue and yellow. When these are mixed with each other, they form the secondary colours orange, green and violet. The six tertiary colours are formed thus: by mixing red with orange to make red/orange; orange with yellow to produce gold; yellow with green to produce lime green; green with blue to produce turquoise; blue with violet to produce indigo; and violet with red to produce magenta. We can obtain lighter shades by adding white, and darker shades by adding black. As well as these 12 core colours, I also use the shades pink, amethyst, silver and pearl.

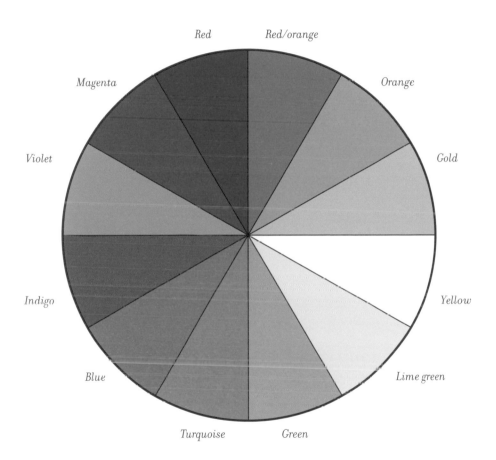

Red   Red/orange   Orange   Gold   Magenta   Violet   Yellow   Indigo   Lime green   Blue   Turquoise   Green

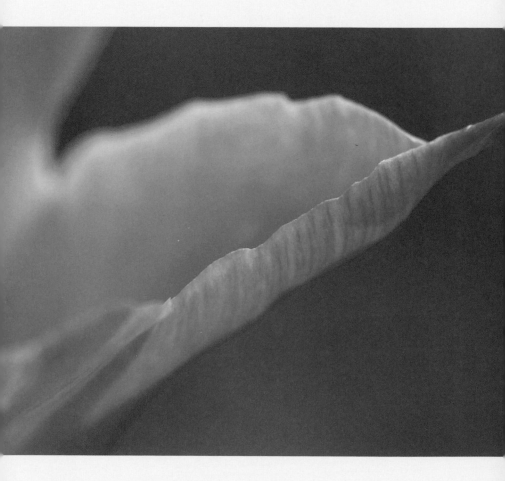

COLOUR AND COMPLEMENTARY COLOUR

Complementary pairs of pigment colours are those which, when mixed together in equal proportion, produce grey. With coloured light, such a mixture would produce white. A colour's complementary is found directly opposite it on the 12-colour wheel (see page 37). For example, the complementary of indigo is gold.

Try perceiving this phenomenon for yourself by staring fixedly at a square of coloured paper until a halo of light appears around it. Then transfer your gaze to a white surface and you will see the complementary colour appear as an after-image.

In therapy, the treatment colour is used in tandem with its complementary colour. It is as if the complementary colour "fixes" the treatment colour. This dualistic approach respects our own dualistic nature, which shows itself, for example, in the interplay between the two sides of the brain – the intellectual left side and the creative right side. To make ourselves whole we should work equally with both aspects of our duality.

GENERAL COLOURS, TREATMENT COLOURS AND THE OVERALL COLOUR

My therapeutic method uses colour in three ways. The names I give these three categories are general colours, treatment colours and the overall colour.

The **general colours** are those to which specific parts of the body vibrate naturally and are, with a few exceptions, determined by the dominant colour of the nearest chakra (see pages 27–29). A general colour is used to revitalize the part of the body that corresponds to the colour's vibratory rate, or to treat energy blocks in that specific part of the aura.

The **treatment colours** are those used to treat particular diseases. Although each disease has its own recognized treatment colours, there will always be a small percentage of people who need to be treated with a different colour. This principle also applies in conventional medicine. The antibiotic usually recommended for a certain disease may be effective in, say, 95 per cent of cases, but for the remaining five per cent a doctor will need to prescribe another antibiotic. What suits one person may not necessarily suit another. In cases when the prescribed colour is not effective, the colour therapist has to listen to his or her intuition, which will often tell them the appropriate colour to use.

The **overall colour** is the one that helps a person to find and work with the cause of a disorder. I have given it this name because it is administered to and treats the *whole* person. Because of the job it does, I feel that it is the most important colour. The overall colour can be administered, with its complementary, by treating the entire body with the colour therapy instrument (see pages 84–85). If a therapist is using contact healing (see page 82), he or she can administer the colour just through the soles of the feet, because the feet are a microcosm of the whole body. You can also administer the overall colour to yourself by using techniques such as visualization, meditation and colour breathing (see pages 112–117). Because the overall colour changes as you start working on yourself, you shouldn't normally use it for more than seven days at a time.

There is a light that shines beyond all things on Earth,
beyond the highest, the very highest heavens.
This is the light that shines in your heart.

THE *UPANISHADS*

(8TH–4TH CENTURY BC)

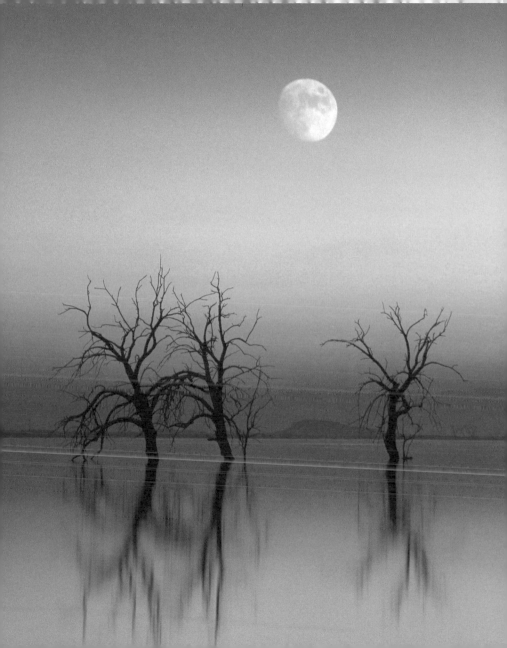

Chapter Two

colours and their attributes

As well as being itself contained within the electro-magnetic spectrum of colours from red to violet, each colour contains its own internal spectrum, which ranges from the palest to the darkest shades. Bright, clear shades tend to denote positive qualities. When they are present in a person's aura, they indicate that he or she is in a healthy and balanced condition. It is the bright shades that we use in colour therapy, in order to promote the benefits associated with them. Dull, muddy shades suggest negative qualities. When these appear in the aura they can indicate physical disease, emotional turmoil or mental unrest. For example, a vibrant green in the aura shows a stable and relaxed state, but a dark, gloomy green may point to avarice or envy. When we select the right colours to resolve particular problems, the muddy shades transform into bright, clear tones.

This chapter sets out the key attributes of the colours to be found on the 12-colour wheel (see pages 36–37), as well as other important therapeutic hues, such as rose pink and silver. We will see how each of these colours affects us physically, what it may indicate when it appears in our aura, and some of the symbolism associated with the colour. This knowledge helps us to choose the best colours for keeping body, mind and spirit in peak condition.

RED AND RED/ORANGE

Red has exciting and stimulating qualities, but it also has the ability to constrict. It is, therefore, not a good colour for asthmatics. The colour is linked with the heart and blood and so it is associated with love, life and sexuality. Exposure to red light quickens the heart rate, increases blood circulation and prompts the release of adrenaline (epinephrine), making it a colour that should be used with caution on those with heart problems such as high blood pressure. Red increases the blood supply to infected parts of the body and so helps to accelerate the healing process. Emotionally, red can cause us to become aggressive and argumentative.

In the aura, a clear, bright red suggests generosity, ambition and affection; dark red indicates courage, deep passion, hatred and anger; a reddish brown shows sensuality; a cloudy red points to greed and cruelty.

Combining the masculine and feminine energies of red and orange respectively, red/orange brings a sense of wholeness and harmony.

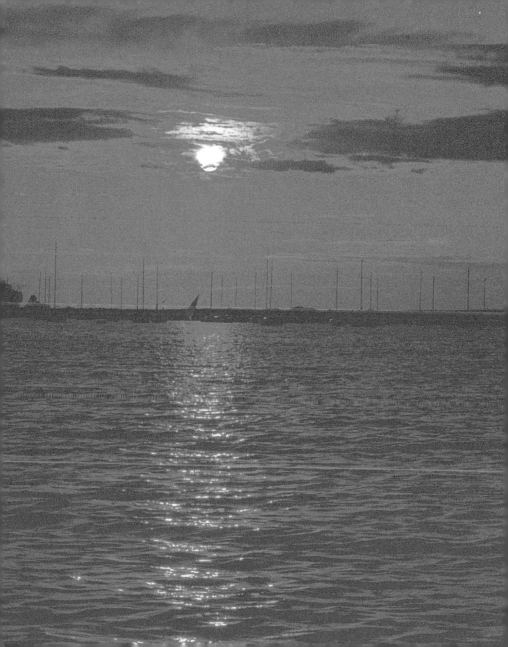

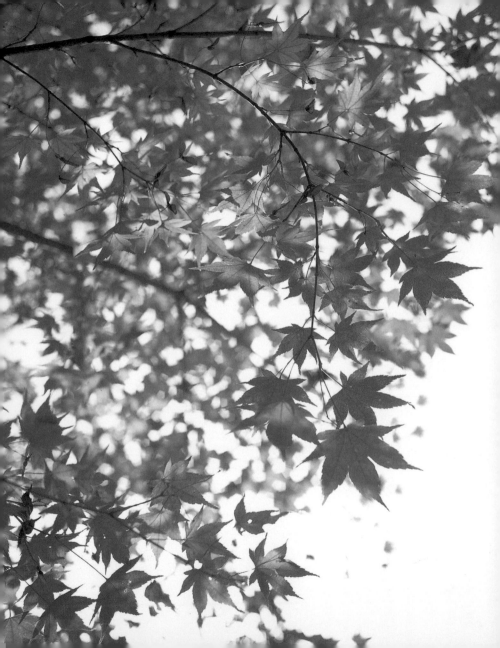

ORANGE

Orange appears next to red on the colour spectrum, making it a warm colour but without the vibrant heat of the red ray. Being associated with feminine energy, it is more gentle than the stimulating, masculine energy of red, and so it is sometimes used therapeutically – for example, to increase circulation – in cases when red would be too intense. It is the colour of joy and happiness, and helps us to achieve a balance between our physical and mental aspects. Orange gives freedom to thoughts and feelings and disperses heaviness, allowing the body to perform natural, joyful movements.

The vitality associated with orange brings about a change in our biochemical structure, helping us to shake off depression. This makes it a good colour for those who are feeling lethargic or miserable.

In the aura, a bright, clear orange denotes health and well-being; a deep orange, pride; a muddy, cloudy orange, a low intellect. A profusion of orange in the aura shows an abundance of vital, dynamic energy.

GOLD

The colour gold is created by mixing orange and yellow. A warm and lustrous colour, it is associated with mysticism, saints and divinities and it symbolizes universal spirit in its perfect purity.

In Western medicine, the metal gold has long been prescribed (in compound form, either as an injection or as a tablet) for rheumatoid arthritis, as well as for spinal problems and tuberculosis. In homeopathy it is a remedy for depression. Anthroposophic medicine (a spiritual approach to healing developed by the Austrian philosopher and scientist Rudolf Steiner) claims that gold improves circulation, increases body warmth and can also be made into a salve to treat lupus.

In colour therapy, gold energizes the entire nervous system when it is applied to the spine. It also invigorates when it is applied to the spleen and, like yellow, it exerts a beneficial effect on the skeletal system, helping to break up painful deposits resulting from rheumatism and arthritis.

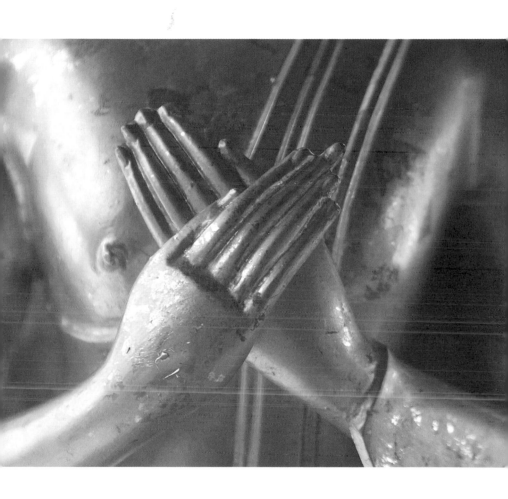

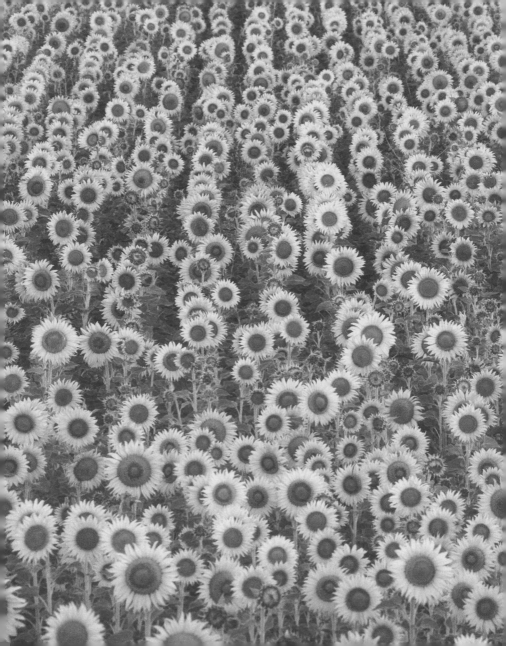

YELLOW

The colour nearest to sunlight, yellow radiates warmth and joy. It also symbolizes the power of the intellect.

Among the physical benefits of the colour is its ability to generate energy in the muscles. Yellow is good for the skin: it improves skin texture and heals scars, eczema and other skin disorders. It is also beneficial for all arthritic and rheumatic conditions.

Yellow is the colour of detachment and can help us move away from obsessional thoughts and behaviour. Because yellow works with the intellect, it is good to use (in small quantities) in places of study. However, to be completely surrounded by yellow for a long period of time could cause a state of emotional and mental detachment. This makes it an inappropriate colour for those suffering from certain personality disorders.

In the aura, golden yellow denotes high-minded, noble qualities; pale primrose indicates great intellectual power; dark, dingy yellow suggests jealousy and suspicion; a dull, lifeless yellow relates to false optimism.

LIME GREEN AND GREEN

Lime green is a combination of yellow and green. When administered through the throat chakra it removes stagnant energy from the bloodstream and the etheric layer of the aura. It can also detoxify the livers of those taking powerful medicines or whose diet consists mainly of processed foods (although, of course, an improved diet would be the best long-term measure).

Green provides a sense of balance in all aspects of our selves. It is a very restful colour for the eyes, and so it can be of great benefit if you spend long periods working with computers or under artificial light.

In the natural world, green is both the colour of life, found in the new foliage of spring, and of decay, found in rotting vegetation. It is reputed to cool the blood and animate the nervous system.

In the aura, light green indicates prosperity and success; mid-green, adaptability and versatility; clear green, sympathy. Dark green is the colour of deceit; olive green, of treachery and double nature.

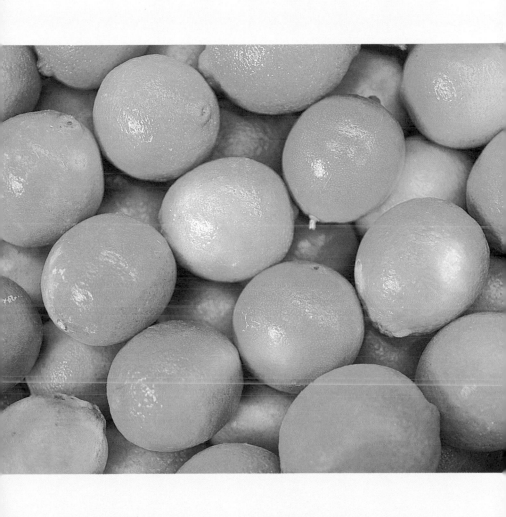

Mere colour, unspoiled by meaning,
and unallied with definite form, can speak
to the soul in a thousand different ways.

OSCAR WILDE

(1854–1900)

The purest and most thoughtful minds
are those which love colour the most.

JOHN RUSKIN

(1819–1900)

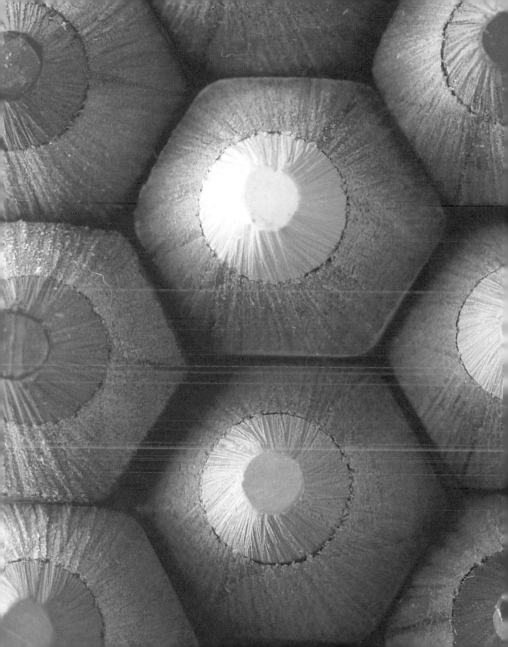

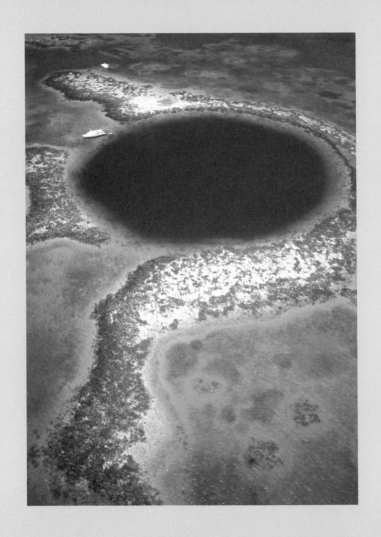

TURQUOISE

Turquoise is the first colour to appear at the cold end of the spectrum. The colour is obtained by combining blue and green and can veer toward either, depending upon the proportions used.

Turquoise was the national colour of Persia (now Iran), possibly because the region houses some of the oldest and finest turquoise gemstones. The ancient Persians believed that the turquoise exerted a strong protective power and used it to ward off evil. The Persian word for these gemstones is *piruseh*, meaning joy.

As well as the major chakras (see pages 27–29), we have 21 minor chakras connected with the physical body. One of these is associated with the thymus gland and radiates the colour turquoise. The thymus gland forms part of our immune system, which makes turquoise a good immunity-boosting colour. Because it is a cooling shade, turquoise can soothe inflammatory conditions, especially when it is used in conjunction with its complementary colour, red/orange.

BLUE

Also situated at the cold end of the spectrum, next to turquoise, blue is the colour of inspiration, peace and tranquillity. It is, therefore, an excellent colour to use as a focus for meditation and in places of healing, where patients need a restful environment in which to recuperate. In direct contrast with red, blue gives the impression of expansiveness: a blue-painted room will seem larger than it really is.

Blue is associated with sadness and depression — hence we describe ourselves as "feeling blue". Clearly, then, it is not a good colour to use if you are depresssed, but it can provide relief to sufferers of many other conditions, including asthma, stress, insomnia and high blood pressure.

In the aura, a deep, clear blue represents pure religious feelings; a pale, ethereal blue indicates devotion to a noble idea; bright blue suggests loyalty and sincerity. A predominance of blue in the aura signifies an artistic, harmonious nature, and spiritual understanding.

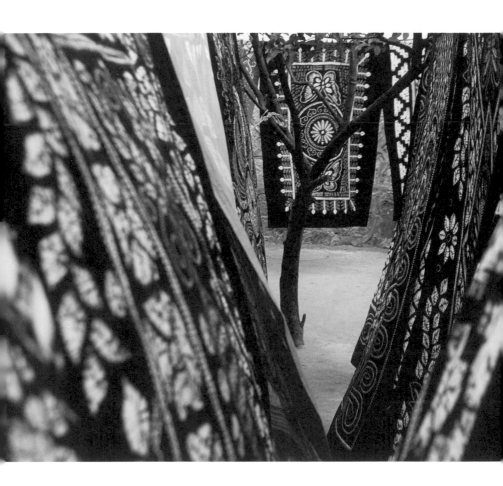

INDIGO

Indigo comprises blue and violet and was originally obtained from the indigo plant. Producing the dye was a lengthy and costly business, which made it extremely rare until the advent of synthetic dyes.

Indigo can create an impression of infinite space and time and can bring about the conditions required for self-reflection and contemplation. Its association with the brow chakra helps foster transcendent vision and an ability to hear the voice of our own intuition.

The indigo ray is cold and astringent and has the capacity to induce anaesthesia in the physical body. This makes it a very powerful painkiller. It is also a colour that helps to purify both the blood stream and the psychic currents found in the aura. Used therapeutically it can relieve tension, muscular strains, neuralgia and insomnia. It can also be employed to treat nosebleeds.

Like the colour blue, indigo can intensify depression in a person already suffering from this condition, so it should be used with caution in these circumstances.

VIOLET

Violet, a mixture of red and blue, has the shortest wavelength and highest energy of all the spectral colours. In the medieval era, violet dye – like indigo – was expensive to produce, which is perhaps why we associate violet, or purple, robes with royalty.

The psychological effects induced by violet include self-respect, dignity, and depth of feeling. It can lead us into realms of spiritual awareness, helping us to become united with our true self or divine inner being.

Violet can treat psychological disorders such as schizophrenia and manic depression, and, when applied to the heart chakra along with rose pink, it soothes a "broken heart". It also helps to combat diseases of the scalp, as well as viral and bacterial infections.

Violet creates balance between the conflicting energies of its constituent colours: the vibrant, masculine red and the calm, feminine blue. However, the colour does have negative aspects – relating, in particular, to the abuse of power and sexuality for personal gain.

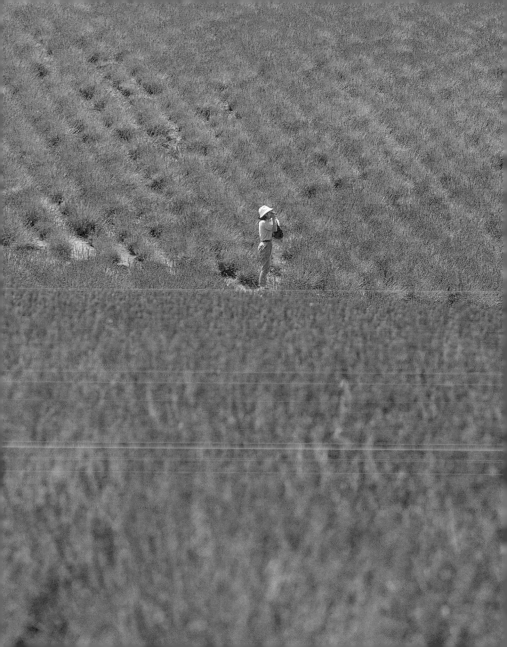

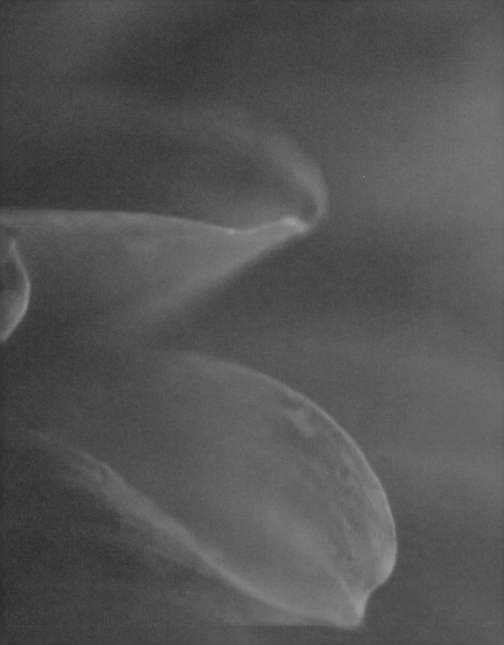

MAGENTA

Magenta is a combination of red and violet. As a dye it was first produced by the French, who called it *fuchsine* after the fuchsia plant. It was renamed magenta by the Italians, after a village in Lombardy that was the site of a particularly bloody battle in 1859.

In the 1930s a bright, strong, intense magenta was called "shocking pink". In the 1950s, a similarly vibrant tone was known as "hot pink" and in the 1960s as "kinky pink". Names such as these make magenta appeal to some people as an exciting, fun colour, while to others it appears sensuous and voluptuous.

On all levels – physical, emotional and mental – magenta is the colour of "letting go". It helps us to relinquish old thought patterns that we have been conditioned to follow, to release emotions that tie us to the past, and to give up situations, such as an unfulfilling job or relationship, that are holding us back. When we are able to rid ourselves of these impediments, we are truly free to flow with the energies of life.

BLACK AND WHITE

White contains all colours and reflects all light. Associated with innocence, purity and change, it is strongly connected to spirituality. The spiritually adept describe being able to "see" and to merge with the white light of God-consciousness.

In colour therapy, the practitioner can use white light when he or she is uncertain which colour to apply. The recipient will then take from that light the colour needed to return them to a state of balance.

Black is not used in healing: it absorbs everything into itself (which is why wearing black in summer makes us feel hotter). It is generally seen as a negative colour associated with pessimism and evil. However, black can be viewed more positively – as the sacred darkness of the earth, which nurtures germinating seeds.

Black is white's complementary – the two colours represent Alpha and Omega, the beginning and the end. We start in the darkness of ignorance and slowly, with conscious effort, walk into the light of understanding.

OTHER HEALING COLOURS

The 12-colour wheel forms the basis of my colour-therapy palette, but there are some other significant shades that I often use.

Rose pink is a mixture of red and white. Gentle and nurturing, it is associated with well-being, and is useful in therapy when it is felt that red would be too powerful. It is the colour connected with unconditional love and is beneficial for those suffering from a "broken heart".

Silver is related to the moon, and the colour's shiny appearance provides a mirror for our own personality. Colloidal silver (silver particles suspended in water) was commonly used, until the advent of synthetic medicines in the 1930s, for various purposes – particularly as a topical antiseptic for inflammation and burns. Recently it has enjoyed a revival, following biomedical research suggesting that it can also help combat bacterial, viral or fungal infections. The silver ray has cleansing, cutting and burning qualities and is used mainly (and only by qualified practitioners) for cases of obsession.

The colour **pearl** is also associated with the moon, as well as with feminine energy. The American psychic healer Edgar Cayce asserted that pearl activates purity, strengthens the body and stimulates creativity. When the colour is applied to the throat chakra and the spleen, it will break up and disperse blockages or serious disharmonies in the aura's etheric layer. When pearl is applied to the solar plexus, it can be beneficial for abdominal complaints that arise from stress, anxiety and emotional imbalances.

Amethyst is a purple shade named after the stone of that colour. The appearance of amethyst in the aura indicates a spiritual orientation. In healing, the colour is used to give both spiritual and physical strength. It is applied to the heart centre as a treatment for heart disease and to remedy cases of embitterment or hatred, and – in tandem with rose pink – to help mend a "broken heart". Amethyst heals the heart, and rose pink fills it with unconditional love. In ancient Greek, *amethyst* means "not drunk" – the stone was reputedly worn as a protection against liquid overindulgence!

visiting a colour therapist

There are many ways in which you can access the benefits of colour therapy yourself to deal with minor ailments or to promote general well-being (as we shall see in Chapter Four). However, you may also wish to visit a qualified colour therapist, particularly if you are suffering from a more serious complaint. In this chapter, we will look at what you are likely to encounter in a colour therapy treatment session.

Methods vary with individual practitioners, but in every case the object of the treatment is to channel the appropriate healing colours into the patient. As with any form of therapy, the first step is to gain as deep an understanding as possible of your problem or problems. Then we establish the overall colour – the one that will most help you to discover and address the underlying cause of your complaint. There are various methods of finding the overall colour, including dowsing and kinesiology (see pages 78–81).

The next step is to administer the colour. Sometimes this is performed in a visible way – for example, by shining coloured light. But some colour therapists choose to transmit colour through their hands. At the Oracle School, where I practise, we do both – the former by using a colour therapy instrument (see pages 84–85) and the latter by means of contact healing (see page 82).

WHAT TO EXPECT

Responses to colour treatment vary. Some people are able to feel the vibrational energies of the colours being administered; others report actually "seeing" the colours when they close their eyes. Reaction to colour is, I believe, based largely upon a patient's degree of sensitivity. However, if you can't see or feel the colours it doesn't mean that the treatment hasn't worked.

Because colour affects the whole person and not just your symptoms, you may become very emotional during and after a treatment, as underlying issues rise into your conscious mind. For some patients this can be so upsetting that they decide to call a halt to the treatment. Working with the overall colour between treatments can also initiate changes in your emotional state – again an indication that you're having to deal with hitherto suppressed feelings. Because these issues may well be the root cause of your problem, it's important to face them. In this respect your therapist's counselling skills are of the utmost importance.

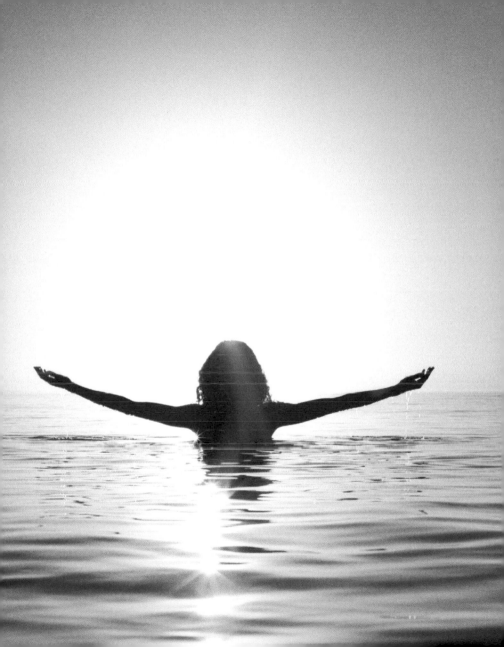

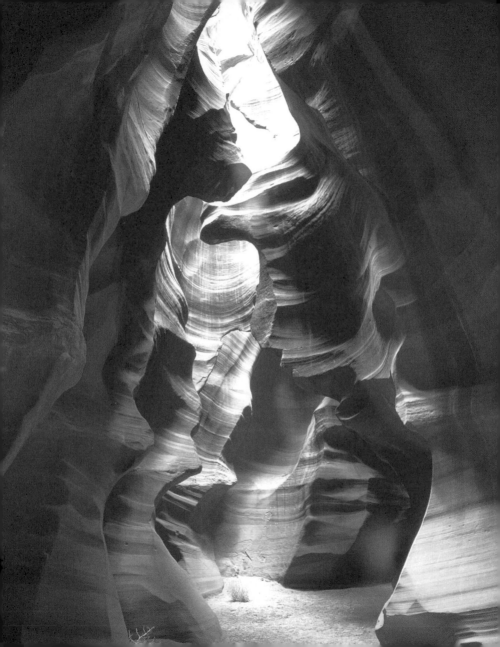

Look within! The secret is inside you!

HUI NENO

(638-713)

Feeling is deep and still; and the word
that floats on the surface
Is as the tossing buoy, that betrays
where the anchor is hidden.

HENRY WADSWORTH LONGFELLOW

(1807-1882)

FINDING THE OVERALL COLOUR

At the Oracle School of Colour, we choose from three methods – kinesiology, dowsing and the spinal diagnostic chart – to find a person's overall colour (see page 41).

Kinesiology is a muscle-testing procedure designed to determine the imbalances within a person, the cause of the imbalances, and the most effective treatment for them. The technique is often used to test for food sensitivities: a minute amount of each food to be tested is placed on the tongue and then the kinesiologist assesses either the legs or the arms. If they feel weak when gentle pressure is applied, it is an indication that the person is allergic to, or intolerant of, the food in question.

The same principle applies when using kinesiology to find the overall colour. A colour therapist will first test your muscle tone by gently pressing down on your outstretched arm. He or she will then ask you to resist the applied pressure. Finally, they will ask you to face the light and to hold up to your eyes silk or cotton fabrics or coloured light filters (known as gels) in the colours of the 12-colour wheel (see pages 36–37). As you look at each colour, the therapist will press on your arm – if your arm feels weak then it is an indication that you are deficient in that colour. If you seem to be in need of more than one colour, the therapist will dowse (see below) to ascertain which of these is the overall colour the one that will be most beneficial in helping you to find and work with the cause of your problem.

Dowsing is a method of divining which harnesses the radiation that emanates from all substances, including the physical body. A skilled dowser is able to use his or her body as a receiver for this radiation. It then flows through their hands into a dowsing device, usually a pendulum or a forked hazel divining rod, which moves in a certain way to indicate the answer to a question. For example, a pendulum might swing in a clockwise direction if the answer to the question is "yes", and in an anti-clockwise direction if the answer is "no". (When learning to dowse, the therapist has to become attuned to these "yes" and "no" movements, which takes practice.) Over time, the dowser's own vibrational energy will flow

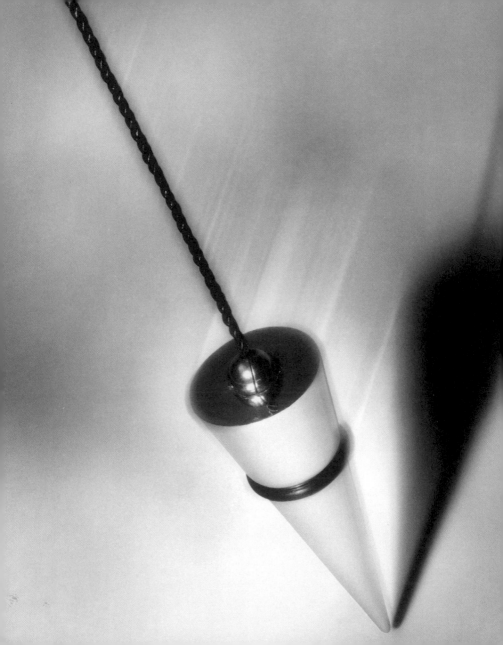

into the dowsing device, making it more effective. It is important, therefore, that they do not let others use it.

To dowse for the overall colour, the therapist holds a pendulum over a 12-colour wheel, with their other hand placed on your arm, to pick up your vibrational energy. They will then ask the pendulum to indicate the overall colour, and it will begin swinging diagonally across two colours – blue and orange, for example. Finally, the therapist will dowse to find out which of the two is the overall colour and which is the complementary.

The **spinal diagnostic chart**, devised by the leading colour therapist Theo Gimbel, is based on the principle that each of our vertebrae relates to a certain aspect of the self (mental, emotional, metabolic or physical) and responds to a given shade of one of the colours of the spectrum. Using a "map" of the spine, the therapist dowses for energy in each vertebra and records the findings on an accompanying chart. This is a complex procedure, but when mastered it is an invaluable tool, not only for ascertaining the overall colour but also for counselling and absent healing (see page 88).

CONTACT HEALING

When administering colour through contact healing, the practitioner's own mind and body become the instruments through which colours are channelled, first into the minor chakra situated in each of their palms and then into the person whom they are treating. The great advantage of this technique is that the therapist can determine the exact shade of the colour. How effective they are as a channel depends upon their sensitivity to colour, the purity of their physical body and their degree of mind control. When channelling, they need to stay focused on the colour and not let the mind wander. The clearer the focus, the more potent the treatment.

Contact healing clears your aura of stagnant energy, applies a variety of colours to balance your emotional, mental and physical aspects, treats chakras that are out of balance and, lastly, administers the overall colour. It involves physical contact, and this therapeutic touch is in itself healing. I personally find this to be the best way of treating with colour.

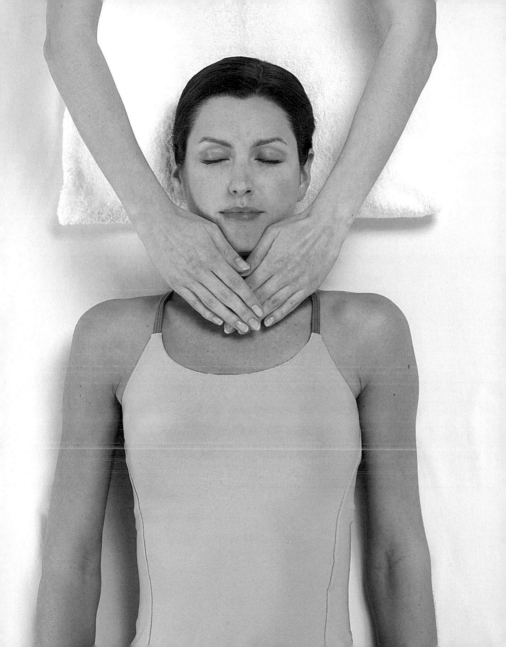

THE COLOUR THERAPY INSTRUMENT

The colour therapy instrument comprises two glass-fronted boxes placed side by side on a table or stand. Each box contains a lamp and has slots into which the practitioner can insert stained glass filters (for the overall colour and its complementary). The boxes are linked to a device that controls both the time of the session and the change sequences between the two colours.

Because light dilutes colour, treatment takes place in a darkened room. The therapist will ask you to sit on a comfortable chair in front of the instrument, and the overall colour and its complementary will be projected over you in turn for just under 20 minutes. The change sequence between the colours is based on the Fibonacci sequence of numbers, named after the Italian mathematician Leonardo Fibonacci (c.1170–c.1250). In the sequence, each number is the sum of the two preceding numbers: 1, 1, 2, 3, 5, 8, 13, 21, and so on. The sequence occurs widely in nature – for example, in the whorls of pine cones and other forms of spiral growth, and in the distances of the planets from the sun. The "golden proportion" established by the Fibonacci sequence also occurs in many aspects of our own skeletal structure: for example, in the relative lengths of the forearm and the hand, and in the positioning of facial features such as the chin, nose and hairline. So, to administer the changes from overall colour to complementary in this way is to apply the colours in the ratio already present in our human form, thereby working in tune with our body.

As we have seen, one of the ways in which we absorb colour is through the eyes, so it is essential that you remove glasses and contact lenses and keep your eyes open throughout your treatment. We also absorb colour through our skin, but coloured clothes interfere with this process – so patients wear a white gown.

An advantage of the colour therapy instrument is that you can actually see the colours, which can be psycholog ically beneficial. It is also invaluable for therapists who find contact healing difficult, or for patients who are averse to being touched. Its disadvantage is that it treats with only the overall and the complementary colours.

Be resolved and the thing is done.

CHINESE PROVERB

The greatest happiness is to transform
one's feelings into actions.

MADAME DE STAËL

(1766-1817)

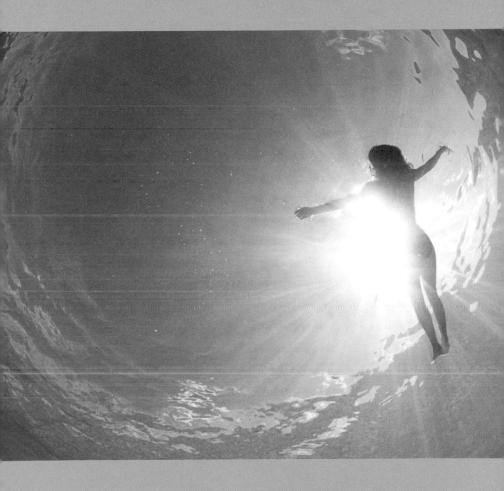

COLOUR THERAPY IN CONTEXT

Colour therapy is extremely versatile. Some therapists even practise absent colour healing, which means that they can transmit colour energies to patients who are not present – perhaps by visualizing the person bathed in a certain colour. Other therapists may ask you to meditate on or to create a *mandala* – a coloured geometric form within a circle, often used as an object for contemplation in Buddhism (see opposite).

What's more, colour can be used in conjunction with many other therapies – for example, sound therapy, homeopathy and counselling. The German scientist Peter Mandel has developed a form of acupuncture that incorporates colour: he calls it "colourpuncture". Mandel discovered that when coloured light is focused accurately on the acupuncture points, it causes powerful healing impulses to be triggered both in the physical and the energy bodies.

For my part, I have researched and initiated the integration of colour with reflexology (see pages 90–91).

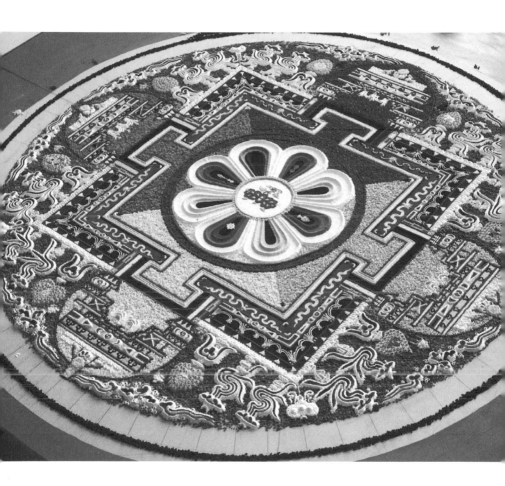

COLOUR REFLEXOLOGY

Reflexology is a touch therapy that treats the whole body through gentle application of pressure to specific reflex points on the hands and feet. These points are believed to be the extremities of the 12 meridians, or energy channels, that carry subtle energy throughout the body. So, in reflexology the hands and feet are the four gateways to the rest of the body.

I discovered that colour enhanced a reflexology treatment and eased conditions that are difficult to treat with reflexology alone. A particular benefit is colour's ability to break down accumulated energy painlessly. And, whereas reflexology focuses on a patient's physical ailments, colour also addresses their emotional and mental issues. I found that when treating someone who was under stress, the application of blue to specific reflexes induced a state of relaxation. It is particularly appropriate to apply blue at the start of a reflexology treatment, because a relaxed body is able to assimilate healing energies more effectively.

The reflexologist applies colour to painful reflexes by means of the "colour reflexology torch". This has a rounded quartz-crystal head and comes with nine stained-glass discs. The head will accommodate two discs at any one time, giving a wide range of colours. When the appropriate coloured disc is inserted and the torch turned on, the crystal head is filled with colour. With the appropriate colour shining, the therapist massages the tender reflex with the head of the torch for approximately one minute, and for a further minute with the complementary colour shining. Reflexes not associated with a physical disease receive the general colour and its complementary (see pages 40–41). The therapist then tests the chakras situated along the spinal reflex of each foot, and corrects any imbalances in them by applying the appropriate colour with the torch.

To end a treatment the practitioner gives the overall colour (see page 41), followed by its complementary, either by means of the colour therapy instrument (see pages 84–85) or by mentally channelling them through the soles of both of the patient's feet.

treating yourself with colour

Colour surrounds us at every moment — we benefit from its healing energies without even realizing it. Walking in the countryside, surrounded by a rich array of calming shades of green leaves and grasses can, when we feel stressed and overworked, help us relax and restore our inner balance. And a beautiful garden, with its palette of flower colours, can be immensely invigorating and uplifting.

In this chapter, you will learn how to harness your innate colour sensitivity in order consciously to enhance your well-being. With practice you will become adept at sensing the colour you need at any given time. Absorbing this colour might involve, for example, the way in which you decorate your home or the clothes that you wear. Wearing specific colours can help us in two ways. First, the garment can act as a filter, allowing colour to be absorbed through the pores of our skin. Second, if we choose a colour that enhances our skin tone, we look good, which can give us a great psychological boost. When we feel happy, our bodies release endorphins, which strengthen our immune system and also act as a natural painkiller.

We will also look at the numerous simple and safe colour therapies with which you can treat yourself. These include colour breathing, visualizing colour, and massaging yourself with colour-"solarized" oil.

THE COLOURS OF NATURE

The colours of our environment affect us in subtle but significant ways. To be surrounded by nothing but dull, drab shades is wearing. However, we can revitalize ourselves by seeking out the living colours of nature.

Carefully examine, for example, the petals of a red rose and notice how each one has its own gradations of tone, which can range from deepest ruby to palest pink. See a tree's buds opening to reveal pale green leaves, which darken as spring turns to summer and flame into orange, gold and brown with the onset of autumn.

Birds, too, can surprise us with the beauty of their plumage, from the irridescent lights in the starling's dark feathers to the exotically coloured "eyes" in the peacock's tail – if you're lucky enough to see one. We can refresh ourselves with the myriad colours and patterns of a butterfly's wings, the markings in the fur of a much-loved pet, the rainbow arcing across the sky … .

Wherever you are take time to admire the amazing colours with which nature beautifies your environment.

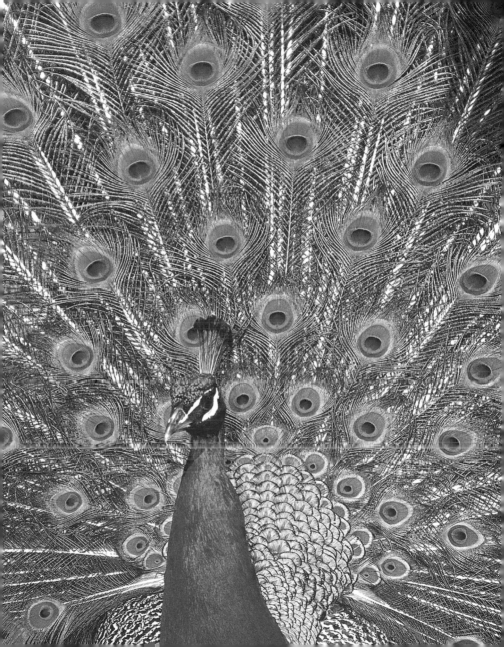

BRINGING COLOUR INTO YOUR LIFE

We bring colour into our lives all the time – through the clothes we wear, the colour schemes we choose for our homes, through our houseplants or the flowers we grow in our gardens. Generally, our choice of colour is based on an unconscious attraction toward it. As you grow in colour sensitivity, however, you will learn to select the colours you need to help keep you in a state of harmony and balance, or to suit the requirements of a particular area of your home.

Injecting colour into your life needn't be expensive. You can achieve it with beautiful coloured scarves or crystals, decorative cushions, lampshades, pictures or posters, or even the pen that you write with. Remember, though, that your colour needs can change on a daily basis. Have you experienced feeling good in, say, a blue outfit one day, but positively disliking it the next? For this reason it's a good idea to have a store of simple, inexpensive objects in a range of colours, so that they can be changed around to suit your requirements.

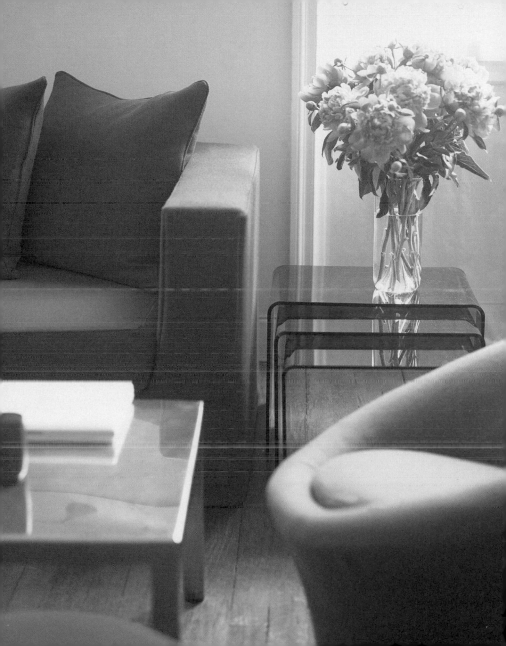

COLOUR IN THE CLOTHES WE WEAR

The colour of our clothes is often symbolic. For example, an Indian bride wears a red sari on her wedding day to denote fertility; the saffron robes of a Buddhist monk symbolize renunciation and humility; the vestments that a Christian priest dons for a requiem mass are black, a sign of mourning.

Often we wear clothes of a specific colour because they flatter our skin tone. However, they can also be worn specifically for therapeutic purposes. To relieve a sore throat, you can wear a red cotton or silk scarf around your neck. Red increases the blood supply, with its infection-fighting white corpuscles, to the affected area. For high blood pressure or stress you could wear a blue shirt, sweater or blouse. If you have a headache, try tying an indigo cotton or silk scarf around your head.

Bear in mind that any clothing you put on underneath the garment carrying the therapeutic colour must be white, because otherwise you will expose yourself to a combination of all the colours you are wearing.

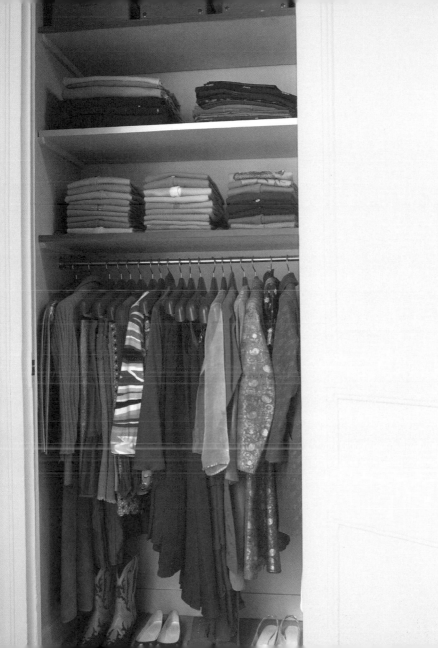

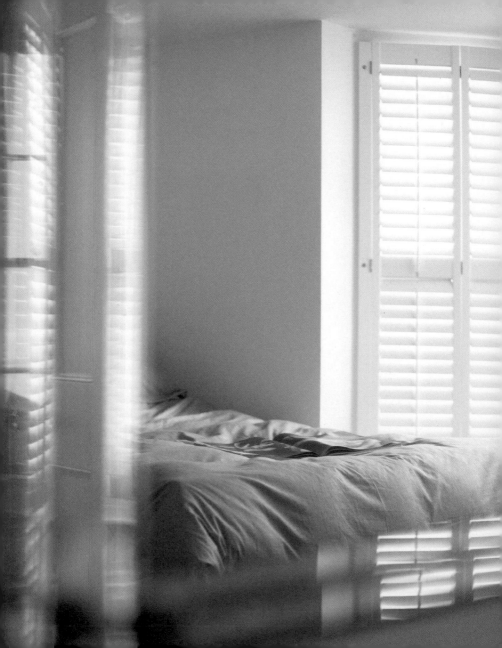

USING COLOUR IN OUR HOMES

A home should serve as a retreat where we are able to revitalize ourselves. The way in which we decorate it is a key factor in deciding the types of energy that we derive from our home. The colours we use should be relevant to each room's purpose, its shape, size, and whether it is sunny or dark. If it's a hot room, choose colours at the cool end of the spectrum; for a cold room, warm colours are best. Dark shades (particularly of red) make a room seem smaller, while pale shades (above all, of blue) enlarge it. Remember, too, that pastels blend harmoniously whereas darker colours tend not to.

A room used for relaxation (for example, a bedroom) would benefit from shades of blue and violet. Orange would be appropriate for an activity room, while yellow accents would suit a study, because yellow stimulates the intellect. Small amounts of red, a colour that aids digestion, could be introduced into a dining room. The hallway is the first part of your home that visitors encounter, so let its colours reflect your personality.

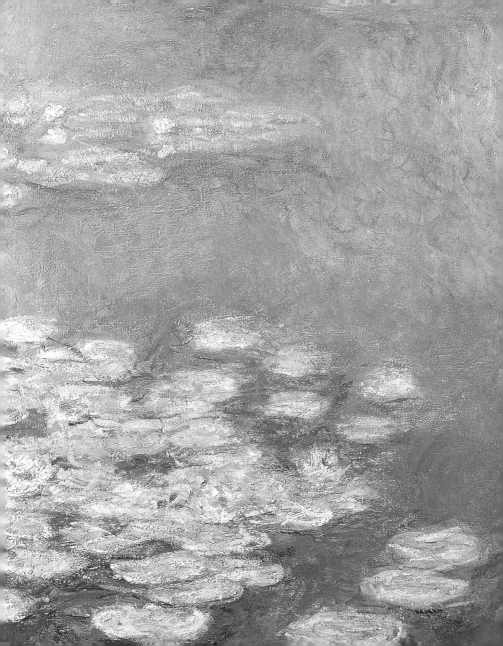

THE HEALING POWER OF ART

There may be times when your colour requirements for a room conflict. For example, if you have a cold bedroom, do you decorate it in a red or orange to make it feel "warmer", or do you exploit the relaxing properties of blue? Displaying well-chosen pieces of art is an ideal way to resolve such dilemmas. Using the example of the cold bedroom, you could paint the room blue and hang a picture painted predominantly in warm colours. What's more, beautiful artworks attract the eye, making them a powerful vehicle for colour.

Even more rewarding is creating your own art. You don't need to have any recognized artistic skills to do this. Making art, no matter what materials we use (paints, crayons, or collages of coloured paper, fabrics, beads, and so on), is a great way to absorb the colours we need to rebalance ourselves — we often gravitate instinctively toward the ones that we are lacking. And losing ourselves in an artistic activity can provide a much-needed release from the stresses of everyday life.

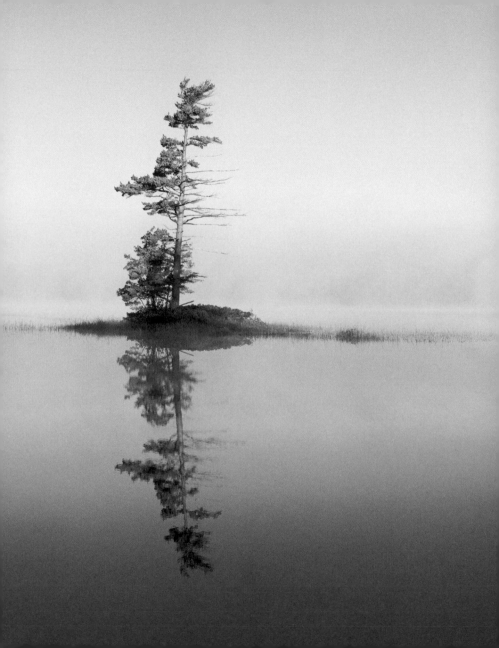

If water derives lucidity from stillness,
how much more the faculties of the mind!

CHUANG TZU

(c.370-300 BC)

The pursuit, even of the best things,
ought to be calm and tranquil.

CICERO

(106-43 BC)

ADDRESSING COMMON AILMENTS

Colour therapy takes many different forms. Some of these – particularly administering coloured light – produce a very powerful effect and should be left to qualified practitioners. However, there are also many gentler, more accessible – but still effective – ways of working with colour that are safe for you to use on yourself to deal with a wide range of common complaints.

The table, opposite, shows some of the conditions that respond well to each of the colours of the spectrum. In many cases the colour and its complementary are to be administered to the whole body, whereas for certain other ailments, such as a headache or pain from an arthritic joint, it is more appropriate to direct the colours to the affected part of the body. Most of the therapies introduced in this chapter can be tailored to achieve this effect. For example, the meditation and visualization techniques on the following pages provide a framework, but you should use your imagination to adjust them to suit your needs and preferences.

COLOUR	COMPLEMENTARY	GOOD FOR:	APPLIED TO:
Red	Green	Constipation	Abdomen
		Cold hands and feet	Hands and feet
		Low blood pressure	Whole body
Orange	Blue	Depression	Whole body
		Head colds	Head
Yellow	Violet	Stimulating the mind	Head
		Osteoporosis	Whole body
		Arthritis	Affected joint(s)
Lime green	Magenta	Toxicity	Liver
Blue	Orange	Stress	Whole body
		Insomnia	Whole body
		Tension	Whole body
		High blood pressure	Whole body
Indigo	Gold	Headaches	Head
		Pain	Affected area
		Making space for oneself	Whole body
Violet	Yellow	Boosting self-esteem	Whole body
		Skin problems	Affected area

WORKING WITH COLOURED MATERIAL

This is a great way to administer a colour evenly over the whole body. The coloured fabric needs to be either thin cotton or thin silk, and long enough to reach from the neck to the toes. If you're working with stimulating colours, it's better to do the exercise in the morning – and just before bed if you're using calming colours.

1   Choose the piece of material you wish to work with. For example, if you've had a stressful day, choose blue material; if you feel depressed, choose orange.

2   Lying in a warm, well-lit room, cover yourself with your chosen colour. This must be placed either next to the skin or over white underwear. Close your eyes and allow the energies of the colour to be absorbed through the pores of your skin for 20 minutes.

3   At the end of this time, before getting up, ask yourself how you feel – be mindful of any emotional, mental or physical changes that may have occurred within you. This exercise can be repeated daily.

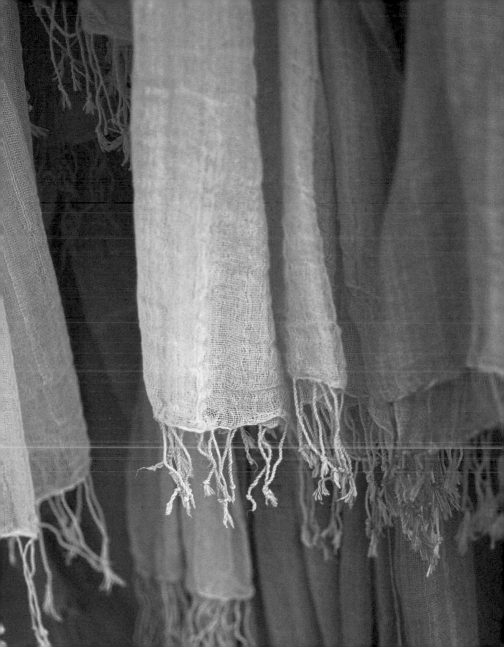

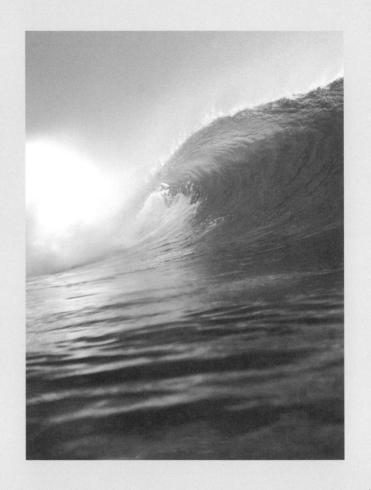

Life's picture is constantly undergoing change.
The spirit beholds a new world every moment.

RUMI

(1207–1273)

All my life through, the new sights of nature
made me rejoice like a child.

MARIE CURIE

(1867–1934)

COLOUR VISUALIZATION

Visualization is an excellent method for relaxing both body and mind. You can use anything from nature as the focus of your visualization – flowers, crystals, leaves, fruit – but each time you work with this method, try to select an object of a different colour, to avoid overexposing yourself to just one or two colours. As an example, here is a visualization for yellow.

1 Lie or sit in a warm place where you can be quiet and undisturbed. Close your eyes and slowly breathe in and out to a count of five until your mind becomes tranquil.

2 Now visualize a daffodil, with its pale outer petals and intense yellow inner petals. Imagine the flower growing until you can crawl inside. Lie down in the flower, resting your head on the stamens. As the sun filters through the petals, you become bathed in a radiant yellow light.

3 Continue to absorb this light for as long as you feel is necessary. Then move out of the flower, open your eyes and take note of how you feel.

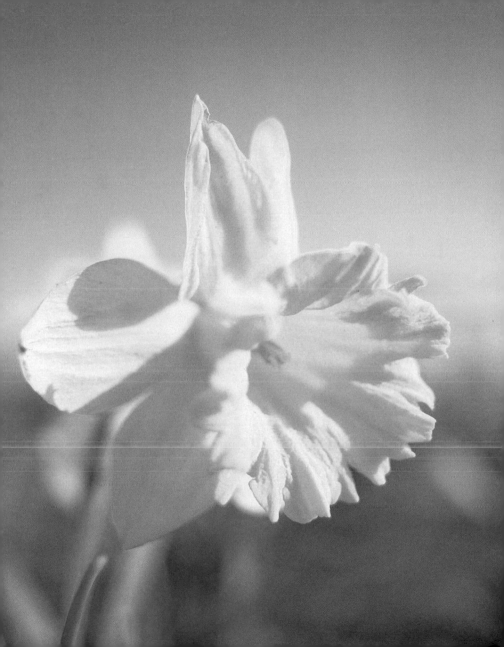

MEDITATION WITH COLOUR

Meditation techniques teach us how to quieten and transcend our thinking mind in order to discover our true self. Meditation needs to be practised in a place free from noise and distraction. Initially, keeping the mind focused may prove difficult, but you will find it easier the more you practise. Each session is complete and unique, so don't try to recapture previous experiences.

1 Sitting in your chosen place, relax your body and mind. Imagine that you are sitting in a glass chalice, similar in shape to a brandy glass. The glass refracts light as it passes through, filling the inside of the chalice with all the colours of the spectrum, which dance around you.

2 Looking up at the rim of the glass, visualize a shaft of white light shining into your crown chakra and over-flowing into the lower chakras. Each chakra takes from the light the colour that it resonates to and, in so doing, becomes energized and clear of stagnant energy. Having recharged your chakras, consider how you feel.

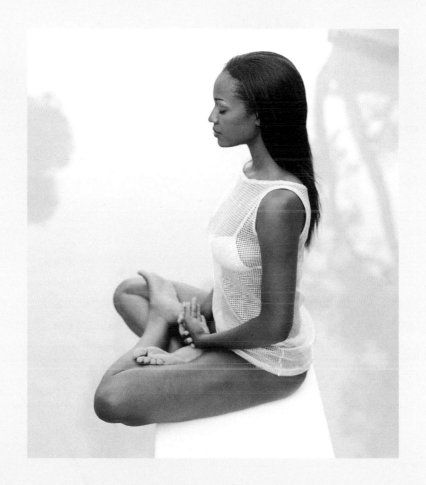

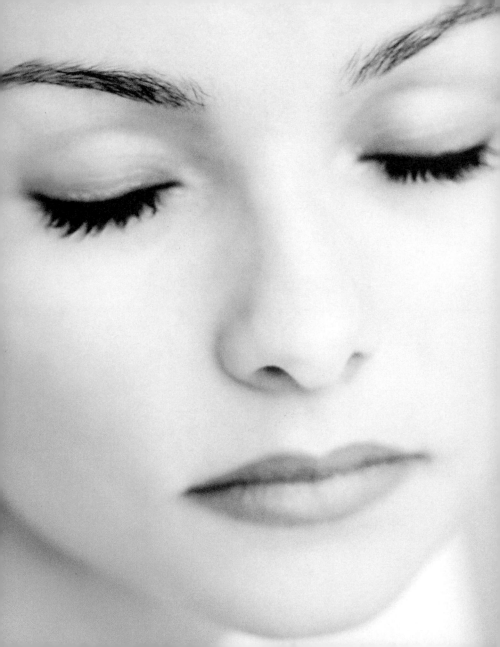

COLOUR BREATHING

Colour breathing involves "inhaling" colour. We can either visualize a colour saturating our whole being or we can direct it to a specific part of the body. Red, orange, yellow, gold and lime green are visualized entering the body through the feet, green through the heart and turquoise, blue, indigo, violet and magenta through the top of the head. Try this exercise for stress relief:

1 Sitting in a warm, quiet place, check that your spine is straight and your shoulders down and back, in order to open your chest. Breathe slowly and evenly.

2 Now breathe into the top of your head a shaft of soft blue light and, as you exhale, visualize this light spreading throughout your body. Each inhalation brings in more blue light and each exhalation intensifies it in your body.

3 After five minutes change to the complementary colour. Inhale orange light through the soles of your feet and draw it up your body with each breath. Breathe in orange for five minutes, then slowly return to your day.

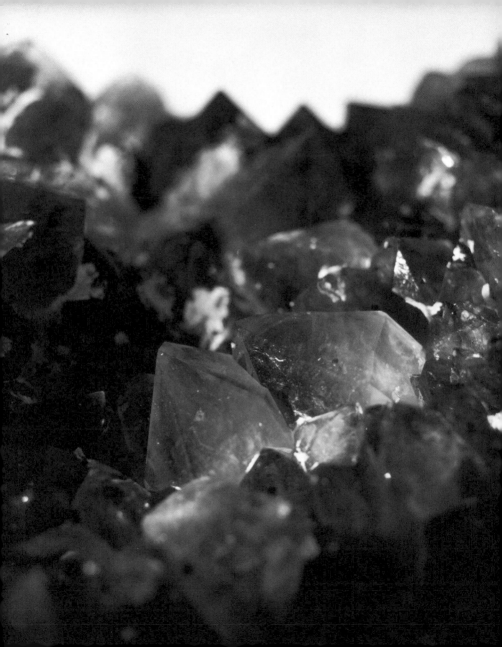

COLOUR AND CRYSTALS

Crystals come in many shapes and colours and they have many uses in healing. Crystals placed around the home will charge with energy the area where they are sited. They will also clear negative vibrations from a room.

In India, gem therapy is associated with ayurvedic medicine, and therapists employ various methods for extracting the stone's colour energy. One method is to burn the appropriate stones and administer the ash to the patient. Another method is to store the stones in alcohol for seven days. This allows the colour's energy to be absorbed into the alcohol, which is then given to the patient in minuscule doses.

Gemstones can also be used to align the chakras. This is done by placing over the chakra a stone of the colour to which that chakra resonates. For example, a ruby or garnet can be used to align the base chakra, which radiates red. A very gentle healing stone is rose quartz. This is especially valuable when placed over the heart chakra of those suffering from a "broken heart".

COLOUR MASSAGE

We can combine the benefits of therapeutic massage with those of colour therapy by using a base massage oil that has been "solarized" with colour. The easiest way to do this is to put neutral massage oil into transparent coloured glass jars with screw tops, replace the caps, and then stand them in a place that receives a lot of light. The jars will keep the oil solarized if left in the sunlight.

The alternative is to put the oil in uncovered opaque white or black jars, place coloured filters on top and then stand the jars in a sunlit place for approximately one hour. To keep the oil solarized, it should then be stored in black jars with black lids.

You can use solarized oil for all manner of problems. For example, indigo oil is good for tense, aching muscles and painful joints; arthritic conditions respond well to yellow oil. For localized problems use the appropriate solarized oil to massage that particular area. If the problem affects the whole body – for example, stress – then the oil could be used for a full body massage.

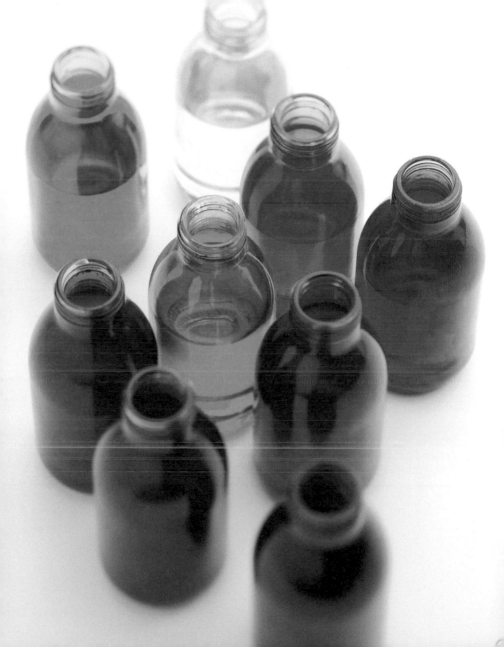

Do not believe a thing because you read it in a book!
Do not believe a thing because another has said so!
Find out the truth for yourself.

SWAMI VIVEKANANDA

(1863-1902)

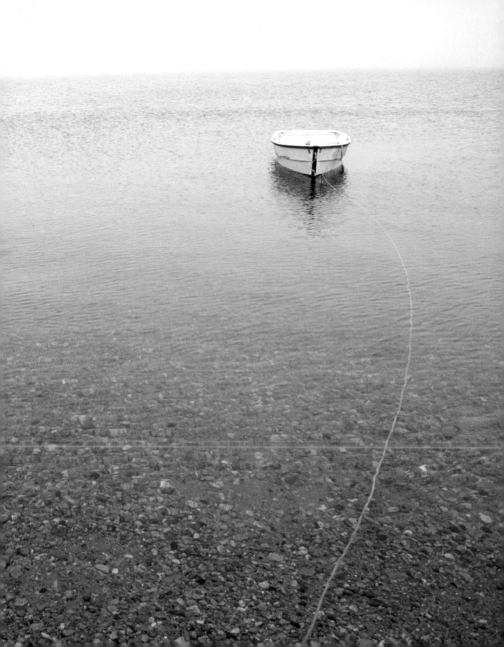

FINDING A PRACTITIONER

If you would like to find a colour therapist, you should choose one who has qualified through an accredited colour school. In the UK, the two regulatory bodies are the Institute for Complementary Medicine (ICM) and the Complementary Medical Association (CMA). Both organizations register only those practitioners who have trained with a school teaching to a required standard. They do not recognize distance-learning courses that contain no attendance modules: a hands-on therapy cannot be mastered by mail. The details of both associations are listed opposite. Contact either or both, asking for the name of a qualified practitioner in your area. The International Association of Colour (IAC) holds a register of accredited practitioners worldwide.

The number of visits you will need will depend upon your state of health and how quickly you respond to treatment. It is usually advisable to attend a minimum of six sessions, but you shouldn't feel obliged to carry on for longer than you deem necessary.

Complementary Medical Association (CMA)

The Falcons, Eagle Heights, Bramlands Close, London SW11 2 LJ

TEL 0845 129 8434   *WEBSITE WWW.THE-CMA.ORG.UK*

Institute for Complementary Medicine (ICM)

Tavern Quay, Plough Way, Surrey Quays SE16 QEZ

TEL 020 7237 5165   *WEBSITE WWW.I-C-M.ORG.UK*

International Association of Colour (IAC)

46 Cottenham Road, Histon, Cambridge CB4 9ES

TEL 01223 563403   *WEBSITE WWW.IAC-COLOUR.CO.UK*

S.A.D. Lightbox Company Ltd

Unit 48, Marlow Road, Stokenchurch,

High Wycombe, Bucks HP14 3QJ

TEL 01494 484852   *WEBSITE WWW.SAD.UK.COM*

Contact the author

PAULINE WILLS, The Oracle School of Colour,

9 Wyndale Avenue, Kingsbury, London NW9 9PT

TEL/FAX 020 8204 7672   *WEBSITE WWW.ORACLESCHOOLOFCOLOUR.COM*

INDEX

Picture Credits

The publisher would like to thank the following people and photographic libraries for permission to reproduce their material. Every care has been taken to trace copyright holders. However, if we have omitted anyone we apologize and will, if informed, make corrections in any future editions.

Page 1 Digital Vision; **2** Getty/Taxi/Franz Camenzind; **3** Image DJ; **11** Getty/Stone/John Lawrence; **14** Corbis/Werner Forman Archive; **20** Science Photo Library/Alfred Pasieka; **25** TopFoto/Charles Walker; **26** Art Archive/British Library; **30** Photolibrary.com/Botanica/Gary Moss; **38** Photos.com; **43** Corbis/Richard Cummins; **47** Photos.com; **48** Photos.com; **51** Photos.com; **52** Corbis/Darrell Gulin; **55** Photos.com; **57** Photos.com; **58** Corbis/Kevin Schafer; **61** Photos.com; **62** Corbis/Keren Su; **65** Photos.com; **66** Photos.com; **69** Photos.com; **75** Getty/Image Bank/Martin Barraud; **76** Corbis/Jim Zuckerman; **80** Corbis/Herrmann/Starke; **83** DBP/Matthew Ward; **87** Getty/Image Bank/Pete Atkinson; **89** Corbis/Geray Sweeney; **95** Photolibrary.com/Ted Mead; **97** Mainstream/Ray Main; **99** Mainstream/Ray Main; **100** Mainstream/Ray Main; **102** BAL/Giraudon (Monet, *Waterlilies*); **104** Getty/Eyewire; **109** Photolibrary.com/Botanica/Nicole Morgenthau; **110** Getty/Eyewire; **113** Photos.com; **115** Getty/Stone/Robert Daly; **116** Photolibrary.com/Hywel Jones; **118** Science Photo Library/Lawrence Lawry; **121** DBP/William Lingwood; **123** Photolibrary.com/Botanica/F Fink Jr Benjamin

Author's Acknowledgments

I thank my sister Patricia Jackson for editorial assistance.